The Vegan's Cookbook

20 Easy Vegan Recipes

Table of Contents

Veganism

Pasta Recipes

Spanish Recipes

Asian Recipes

Pizza Recipes

Soup Recipes

Conclusion

Veganism

Veganism is a strict type of vegetarianism that consists of only plant based products. Veganism excludes all meats and animal products. This means that Vegans do not eat fish, meat, eggs, dairy products, or any of the foods that contain them. Vegans rely on fruits, vegetables, grains, nuts, beans, and seeds. Even though a vegan diet can be very healthy and nutritional, vegans must make sure to eat enough protein, iron, calcium, vitamin B12, and omega-3 fatty acids.

Vitamin B12 is a water-soluble vitamin and is necessary for the production of red blood cells. This vitamin is virtually only present in animal products. This means that vegans have to make sure that they eat foods with added vitamin B12. These foods would include nutritional yeast, fortified soy milk, and fortified cereals. Also, vegans can take a vitamin B12 supplement as well.

Iron is a necessary mineral for red blood cells and the transportation of oxygen in our body. Vegans should make sure to eat dried fruits, dried beans and peas, whole grains, enriched cereals, and dark leafy green vegetables. Also, vegans should try to consume foods high in vitamin C for the absorption of iron. These would be citrus juices and tomatoes.

Omega-3 fatty acids are necessary fatty acids for the brain and the heart. Vegans should eat walnuts, flaxseeds, flaxseed oil, canola oil, and soybeans to obtain those omega-3 fatty acids.

Protein is essential for healthy skin, muscles, and organ health. Vegans should eat foods that are high in protein which included soybeans, soy-based meat substitutes, tofu, soy milk, black beans, lentils, almonds, peanut butter, chickpeas, whole grain products, and other nuts and seeds.

Calcium is an essential mineral for healthy teeth and bones. Vegans should consume spinach, kale, broccoli, blackstrap molasses, collard greens, and calcium fortified products like soy milk, tofu, cereal, and juice.

Lemon Fettuccine Alfredo

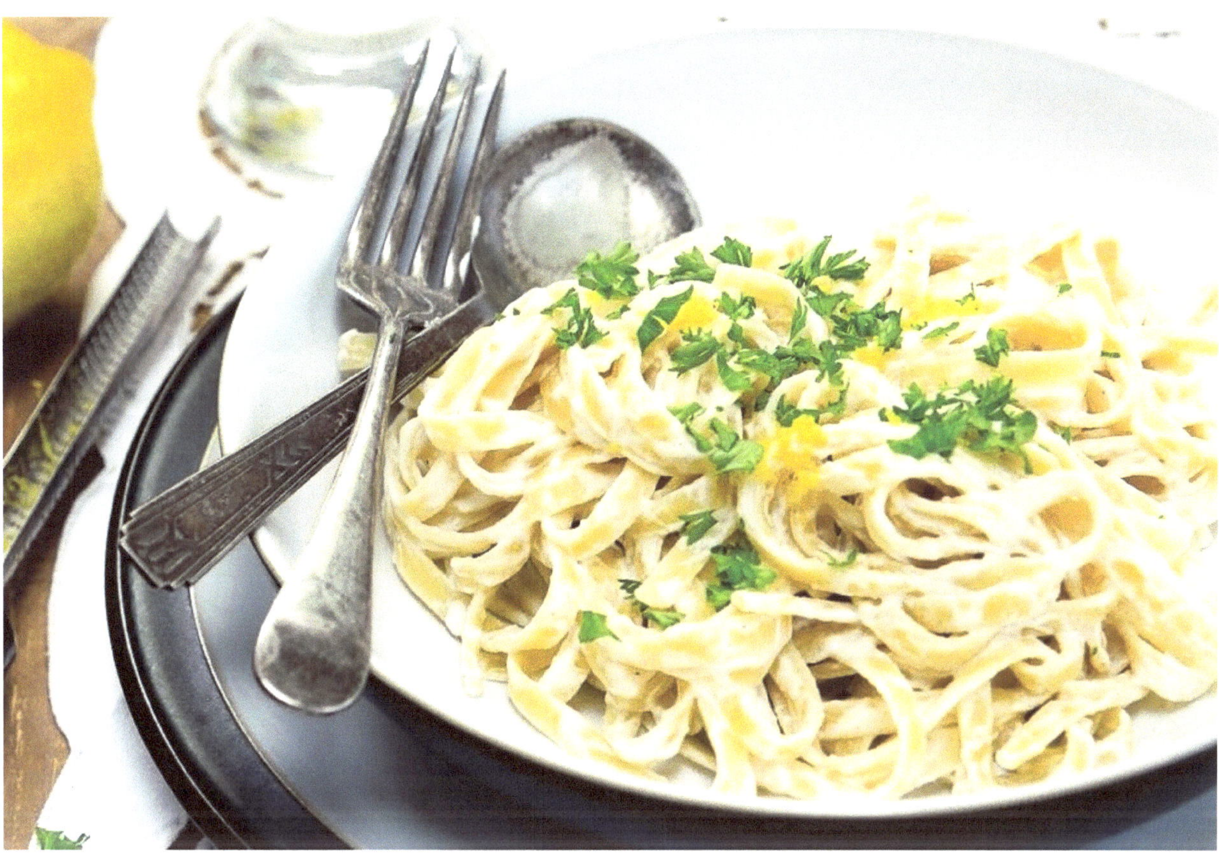

Ingredients

12 Ounces Eggless Fettuccine

4 Ounces Soy Cream Cheese

2 Cups Unsweetened Soy or Almond Milk

3 Tablespoons Nutritional Yeast

3 Tablespoons Blanched Sliced Almonds

1 Teaspoon Finely Grated Lemon Zest

Directions

First, pour some water in a large pot and bring it to a boil. Pour the fettuccine noodles into the boiling water and cook as directed on the package. Afterwards, strain the pasta but keep 1 cup of the cooking water.

Combine the soy milk, soy cream cheese, nutritional yeast, lemon zest, almonds, 1 teaspoon of salt and ¼ teaspoon of pepper into a blender. Blend until smooth,

Pour the oil and some garlic into a large skillet.

2 Tablespoons Extra Virgin Olive Oil

Kosher Salt and Ground Black Pepper

3 Cloves Garlic, Chopped Finely

1.2 Cups Loosely Packed Parsley Leaves;
Chopped

Turn the temperature to medium and stir the garlic until it starts to sizzle. This should take about a minute. Add your blended ingredients into the skillet and bring it to a simmer. Cook until your ingredients are thick and creamy. Add the fettuccini into the skillet and add parsley. Use the pasta water to thin out the sauce if needed.

Finally, you can divide the pasta into four bowls. Sprinkle the top of the pasta with nutritional yeast and dig in.

Green Chili Mac and Cheese

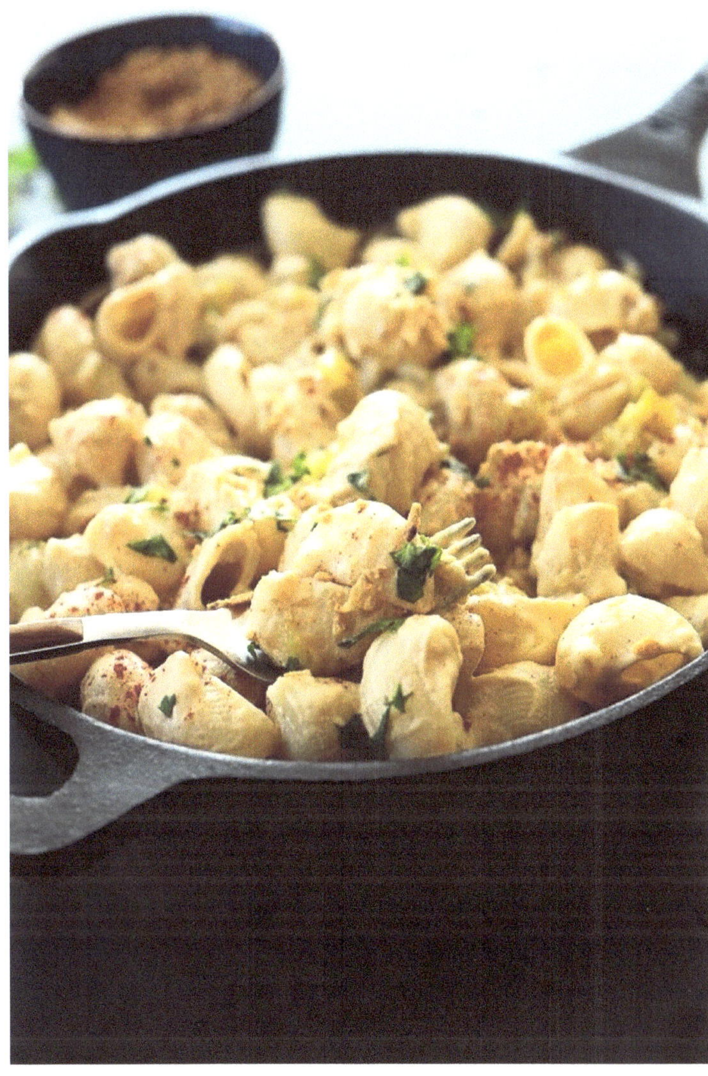

Ingredients

10 Ounces Large Macaroni Shells

3-4 Cloves Garlic, Minced

½ White Onion, Diced

1 Cup Raw Cashews, Soaked for 4-6 Hrs, the Drained

1 Tablespoon Cornstarch

1 ½ Cups Vegetable Broth

½ Teaspoon Cumin

2 Tablespoon Nutritional Yeast

¾ Teaspoon Chili Powder

1-4 Ounce Can Diced Chilies (Half into the Sauce, Other Half for Finished Macaroni and Cheese)

Directions

First, pour the macaroni into a pot of boiling water. Cook according to the package instructions.

Pour some olive oil into a medium size pan. Turn the heat to low. Then, cook the onion and garlic together. Add salt and pepper. Cook until soft for about 7 minutes.

Afterwards, add onions and garlic into a blender with the rest of your ingredients. Only add half of the green chilies. Blend together until smooth and creamy.

Drain the noodles and set them aside for a minute. Add the blended cheese into the pot the noodles were in. Pour the noodles into the pot with the rest of the green chilies. Stir together and serve.

Vegan Avocado Pasta

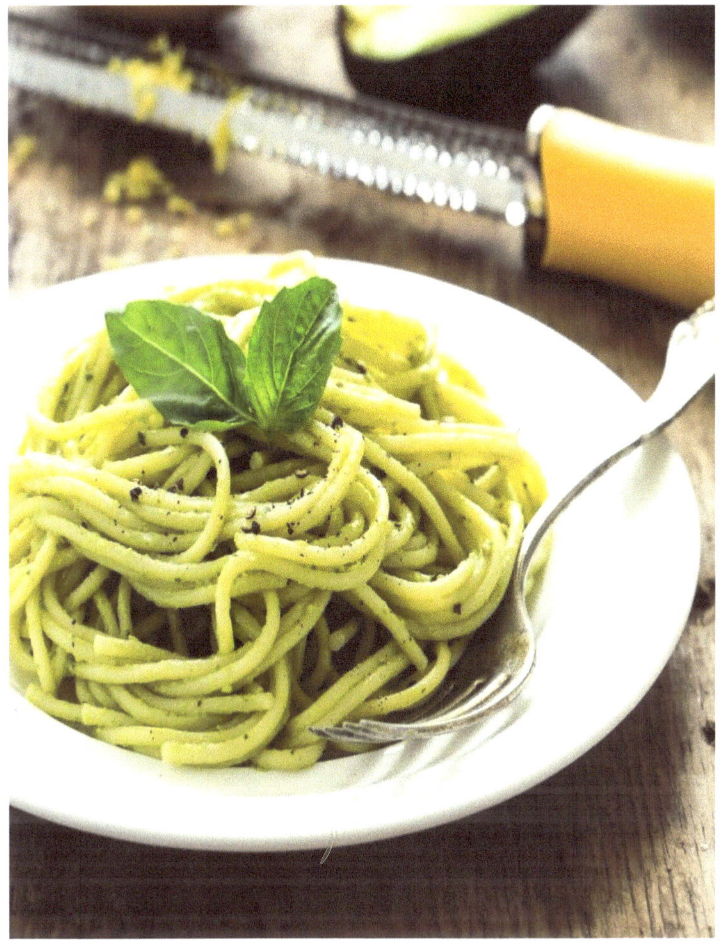

Ingredients

12 Ounces Spaghetti

½ Cup Fresh Basil Leaves

2 Cloves Garlic

2 Ripe Avocados, Seeded, Peeled, and Halved

2 Tablespoons Fresh Lemon Juice

1/3 Cup Olive Oil

1 Cup Cherry Tomatoes, Halved

Kosher Salt and Ground Pepper

½ Cup Canned Corn Kernels, Rinsed and Drained

Directions

First, pour spaghetti noodles into a boiling pot of salted water. Cook the pasta as instructed on the package. Then, make sure to drain the pasta.

Then, combine the avocados, garlic, basil, and lemon juice into a blender. Season it with salt and pepper. As the blender is blending your ingredients, add olive oil slowly.

Finally, pour the spaghetti, sauce, cherry tomatoes and corn into a bowl. Serve afterwards.

Green Olive Pesto Pasta

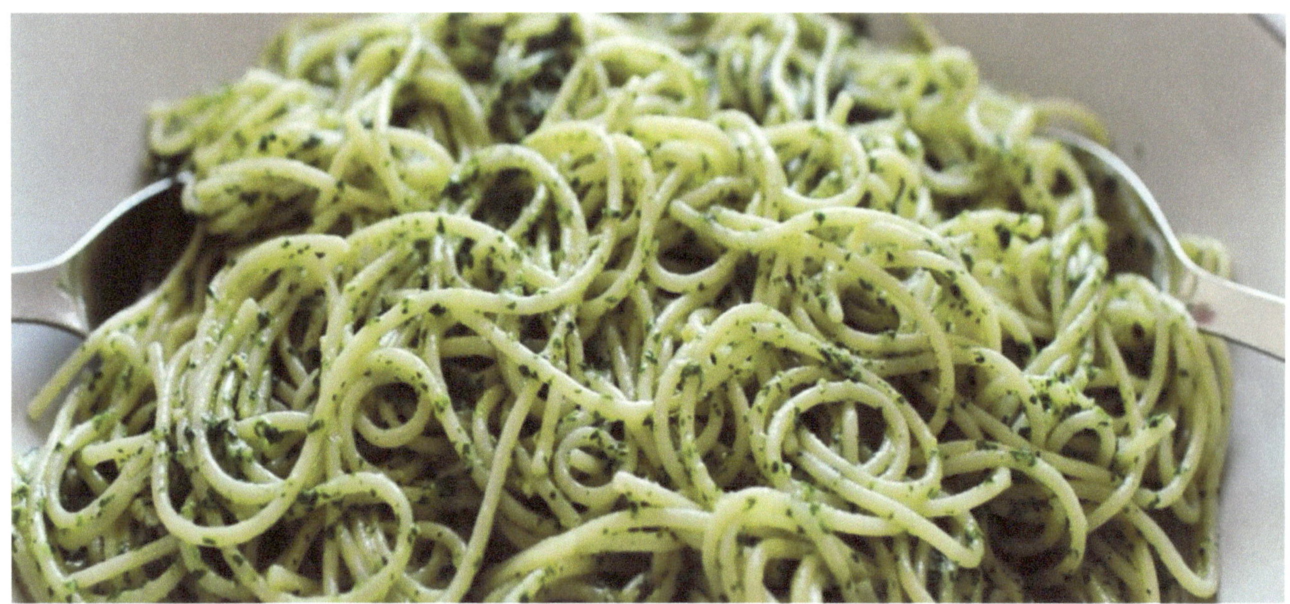

Ingredients

1 Pound Spaghetti

½ Cup Parsley Leaves

¼ Cup Basil Leaves

2 Garlic Cloves, Peeled

¼ Cup Nicoise or Green Olives, Pitted

¼ Cup Pitted Kalamata or Black Olives,
Chopped

½ Teaspoon Kosher Salt

Directions

First, pour your pasta into a boiling pot of water.
Cook accordingly and then drain. Keep ½ cup of
pasta water.

Then, add green olives, basil, and garlic to a
blender. While blending, slowly add the oil.

Then, cook the olive pesto for 2 minutes in a
medium heated large skillet.

Finally, add the spaghetti, the remaining water,
black olives, and salt. Cook until the water is
completely absorbed. Serve immediately.

Zucchini Meatball Pasta

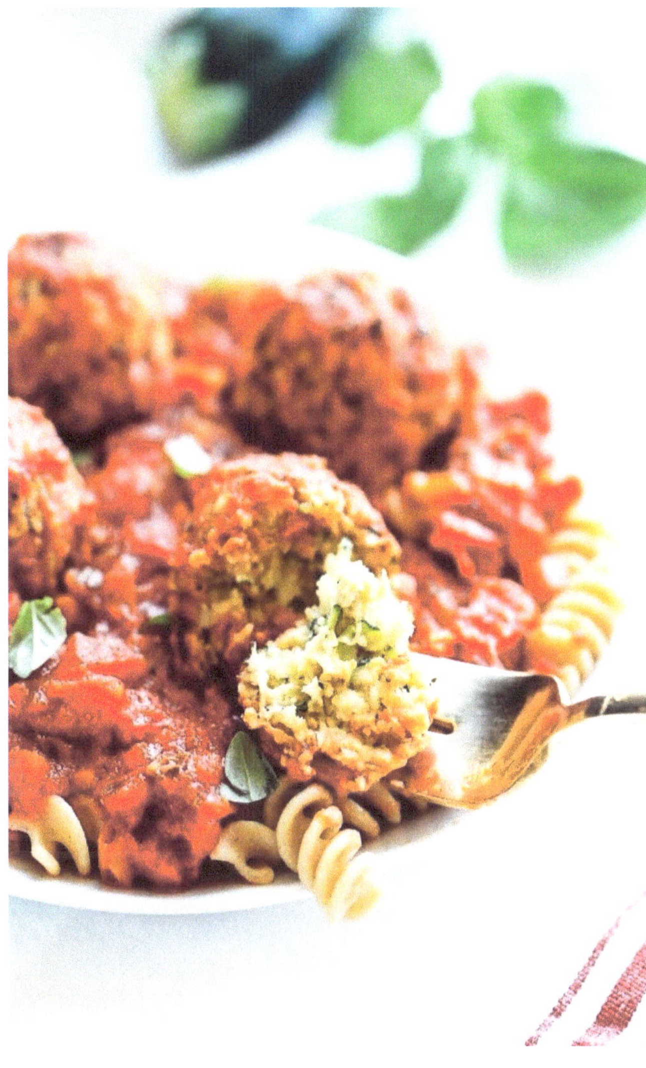

Ingredients

8 Ounces Whole Grain Pasta

15 Ounce Can Chickpeas, Drained and Rinsed

½ Cup Rolled Oats

3 Garlic Cloves

1 Teaspoon Dried Basil

½ Teaspoon Salt

1 Teaspoon Dried Oregano

2 Tablespoons Nutritional Yeast

½ Lemon (Juice)

32 Ounces Marinara

1 Cup Shredded Zucchini

Directions

First, combine the drained and rinsed chickpeas, rolled oats, and garlic cloves into a food processor. Blend for 5-10 seconds.

Second, pour your blend into a bowl with the dried herbs, nutritional yeast, salt, lemon juice and shredded zucchini. Mix your ingredients together and add a little flour if too wet to handle.

Then, preheat the oven to 375°F and apply parchment paper to your baking sheet. Scoop out some of your mixture and roll it into 12 separate balls. Place your balls a few inches apart and then place them in the oven until cooked. They should be lightly golden.

Place your pasta in a boiling pot of water. Cook as directed on the instructions.

Then, drain your pasta and pour your marinara sauce in the pot with your pasta.

Finally, place your meatless meatballs into the pot of pasta and stir. Enjoy!

Portobello Fajitas

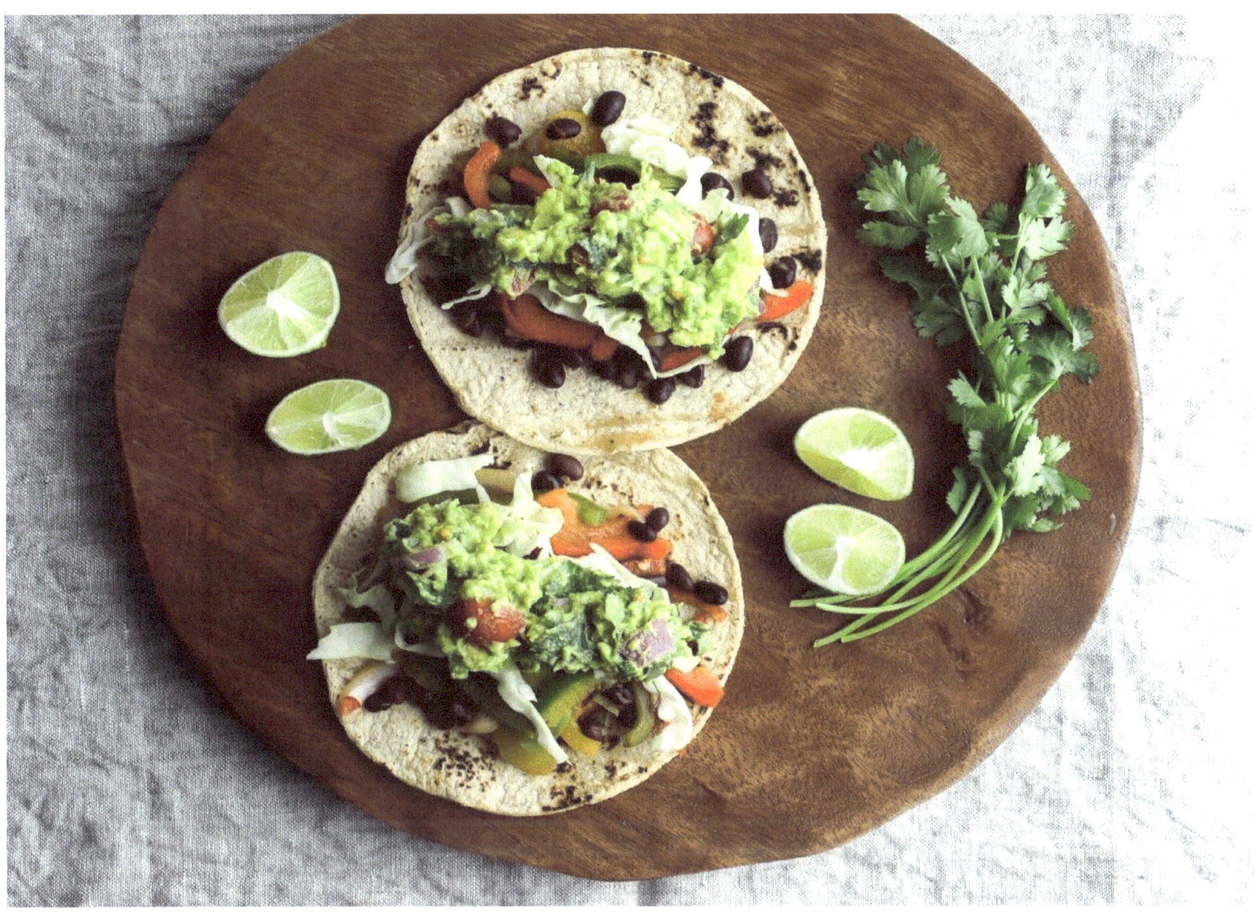

Ingredients

2 Bell Peppers, Thinly Sliced

1 Jalapeno, Thinly Sliced

1 Poblano Pepper, Thinly Sliced

1 Yellow Onion, Thin Rounds

2 Ripe Avocados

4 Baby Portobello Mushrooms, Stem Removed,
Cleaned, Thinly Sliced

Directions

First, heat a large skillet on medium-high heat,
and add some olive oil. Add the onion and
peppers and season lightly with cumin, garlic
powder, and salt.

Then, cook the onion and peppers till
caramelized. Set aside to keep warm.

Heat a medium skillet on medium-high heat. Add
mushrooms and season with a little salt. Set aside
and cover it.

Add 2 avocados to a bowl. Add half of a lime juice

½ Lime (Juice)

Sea Salt

Cumin

Garlic Powder

6 Small Flour or Corn Tortillas

with a little bit of salt. Mix till thick and creamy.

Finally, warm the tortillas a little, place the peppers and onions in the tortillas. Add guacamole or any other toppings to your fajitas.

Veggie Quesadillas

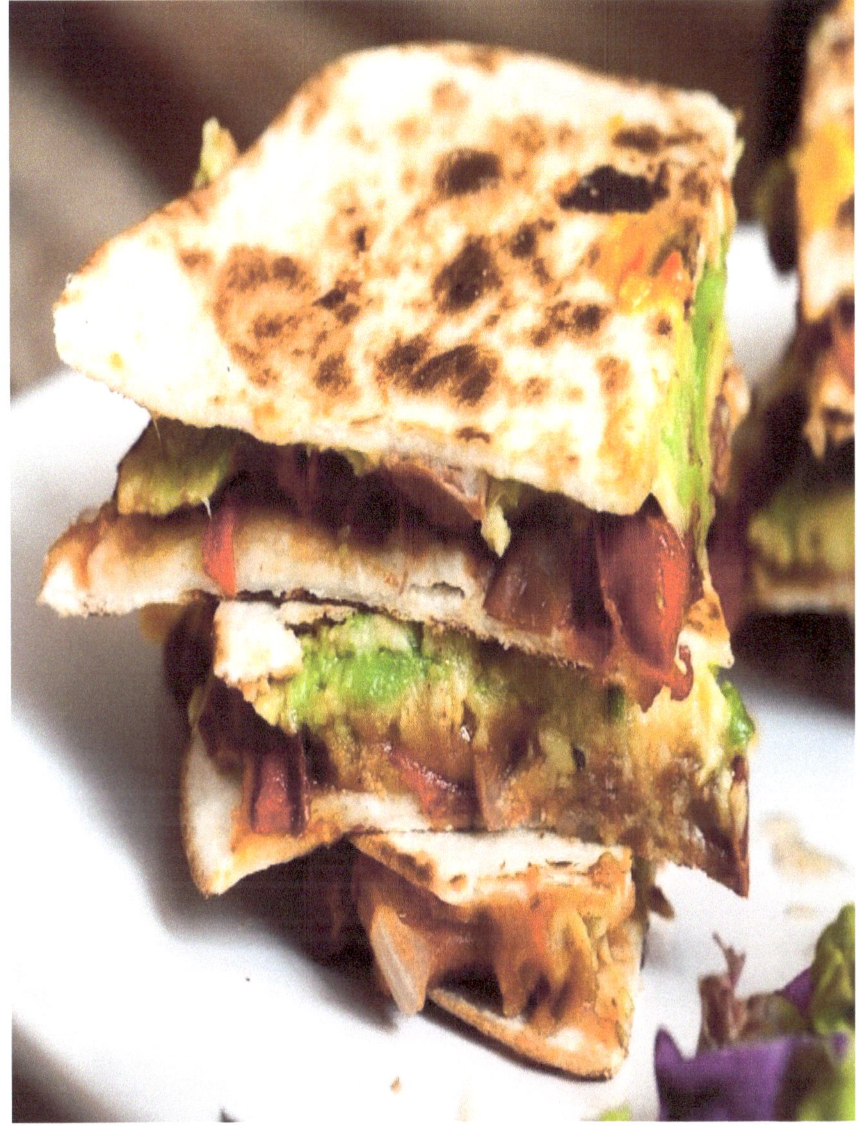

Ingredients

1 Medium Red Onion, Diced

1 Large Green Pepper, Chopped

1 Large Red Pepper, Chopped

1 Can of Black Beans, Rinsed and Drained

1 Jalapeno, Minced or Chopped

1 Cup of Mushrooms, Chopped

1 Teaspoon Ground Coriander

1 Teaspoon Ground Cumin

1 Teaspoon Dried Oregano

3 cups Fresh Spinach, Chopped

Sea Salt and Black Pepper

6 to 8 Brown Rice Tortillas

Directions

First, heat a large, deep skillet over medium to low heat. Add coconut oil, peppers, and onions, and a pinch of salt. Sauté for 15 minutes, but don't let them brown. Cook slowly to get soft and sweet.

Then, add mushrooms, spices, and black beans. Mix everything and continue cooking for 5 minutes.

Add spinach and continue to cook until the spinach wilts. Add salt and pepper and then remove from the heat.

Used a large shallow pan sprayed with cooking spray on medium heat. Place the tortilla shell on the pan and placed some of the cooked ingredients on the tortilla. Put another tortilla on top of your ingredients and allow it to cook. Over time, begin to flip the quesadilla to cook both sides.

Finally, cut the quesadilla in half. Then cut each half into 6 triangles. Enjoy!

Vegan Black Beans and Rice

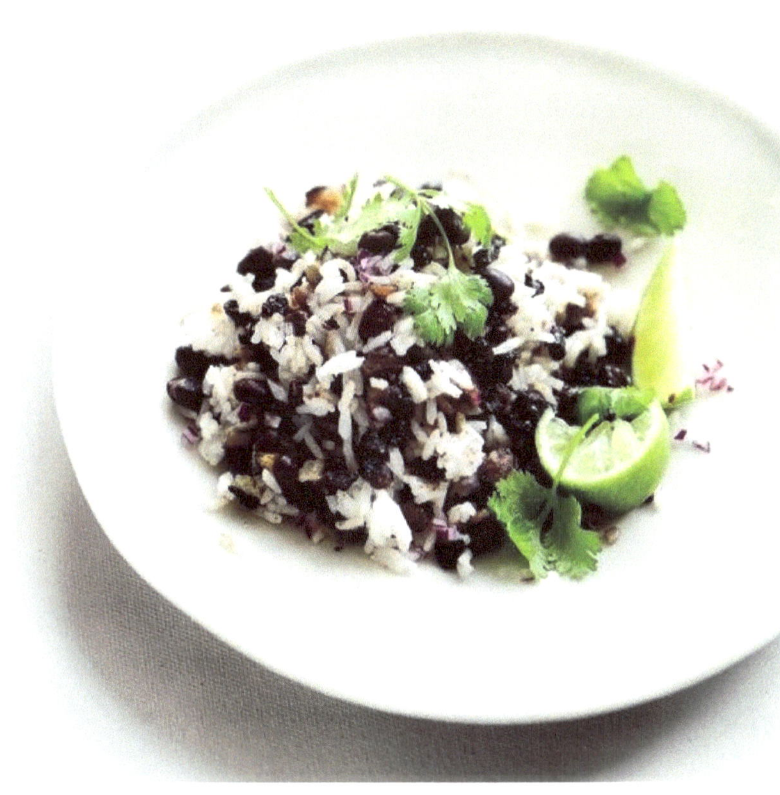

Ingredients

2 ½ Tablespoons Olive Oil

Kosher Salt

2 Cups Long-Grain Rice

1 Large Green or Red Pepper, Chopped

1 Medium Onion, Chopped

2 Tablespoons finely Chopped Garlic

1 Cup Vegetable or Chicken Broth

2 15-Ounce Cans Black Beans, Undrained

2 Tablespoons Red Wine Vinegar

½ Teaspoon Ground Pepper

¼ Teaspoon Ground Cumin

2 Bay Leaves

½ Cup Sliced Scallions (Optional)

Directions

First, combine 4 cups of water with 1 teaspoon of salt and 1 ½ teaspoons of oil in a medium saucepan. Bring the water to a boil.

Second, pour in the rice, stir, cover, and reduce the heat to low. Cook for about 20 minutes or until tender.

Then, in another saucepan, heat 2 tablespoons of oil over medium heat. Sauté the green pepper, garlic, and onion until softened.

Afterwards, add the broth, beans, vinegar, black pepper, cumin, bay leaves, and 1 teaspoon of salt. Cover the saucepan and bring the ingredients to a boil.

Bring the heat to low and let the ingredient simmer for 10 minutes. Remove the bay leaves from the saucepan.

Finally, pour the beans over the rice and sprinkle it with the scallions. Enjoy!

Paella with Red Peppers

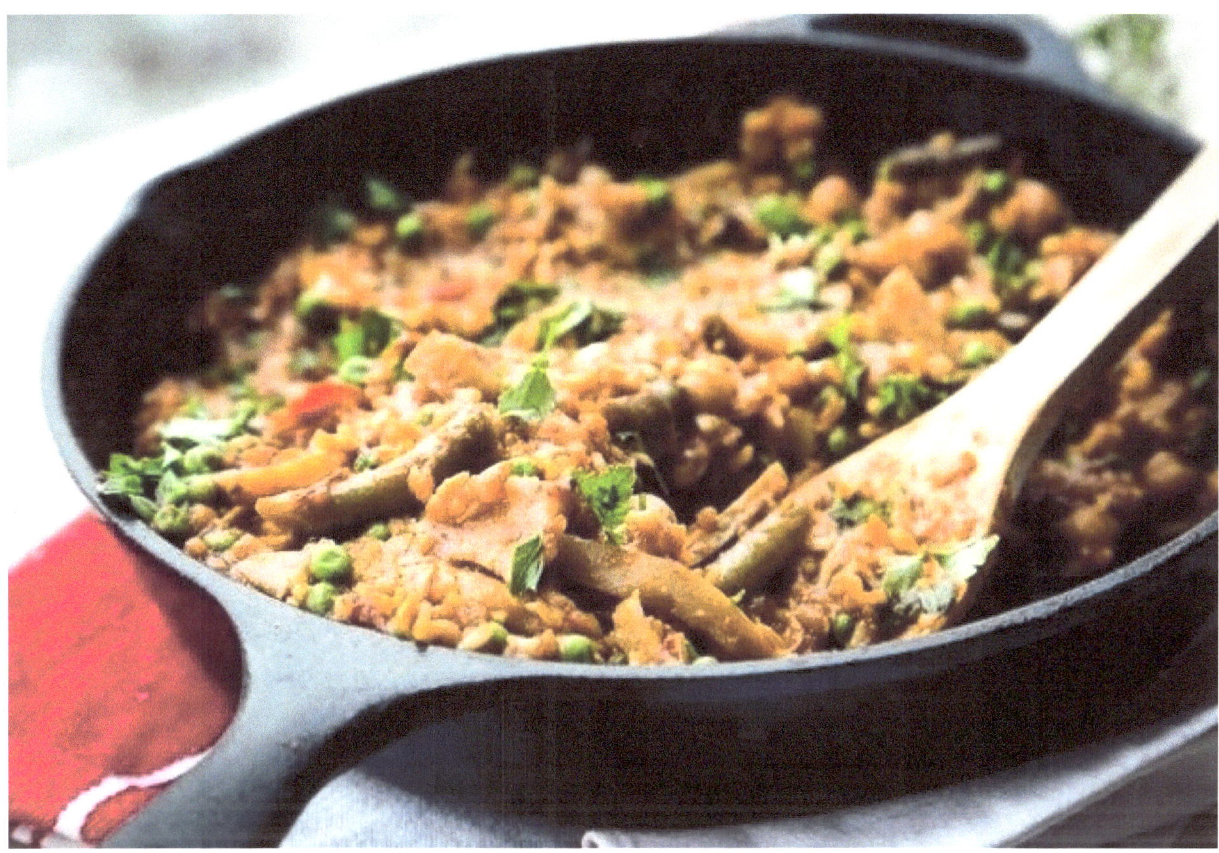

Ingredients

6 Cups Vegetable Broth

8 Strands Saffron

1 Tablespoon Olive Oil

1 Cup Short-Grain Brown Rice

1 Yellow Onion, Diced

1 Yellow Bell Pepper, Sliced

1 Red Bell Pepper, Sliced

Directions

First, pour 3 cups of water and a large pinch of salt into a pot and bring it to a boil. Add the rice and cook for about 20 minutes. Drain the rice and set it aside.

Combine 3 tablespoons of warm water and saffron threads into a small bowl. Set the bowl to the side.

Bring the broth to a simmer, and then keep it at a low temperature.

Afterwards, heat the olive oil in a cast iron skillet. Sauté the onions until soft. Add the peppers and garlic slices. After cooking for about 7 minutes, mix in the tomato paste, crushed tomatoes, hot paprika,

4 Garlic Cloves, Thinly Sliced

¾ Cup Crushed Tomatoes

½ Tablespoon Hot Paprika

2 Tablespoons Tomato Paste

1 Cup Green Beans, Trimmed and Halved

1 Cup Cooked Chickpeas

3 Artichoke Hearts, Sliced

¼ Cup Chopped Parsley

¼ Cup Peas

Salt and Pepper

saffron and some salt and pepper. Let your ingredients cook for a few minutes.

Simmer your vegetable broth. Stir in the artichoke slices, green beans, and chickpeas with the other ingredients. Pour the broth over the drained rice. Let it simmer for a few minutes. Mix the rice in with your ingredients in the cast iron skillet. Cook till all the broth evaporates. Scatter some peas and parsley on the top and then serve.

Burrito Stuffed Peppers

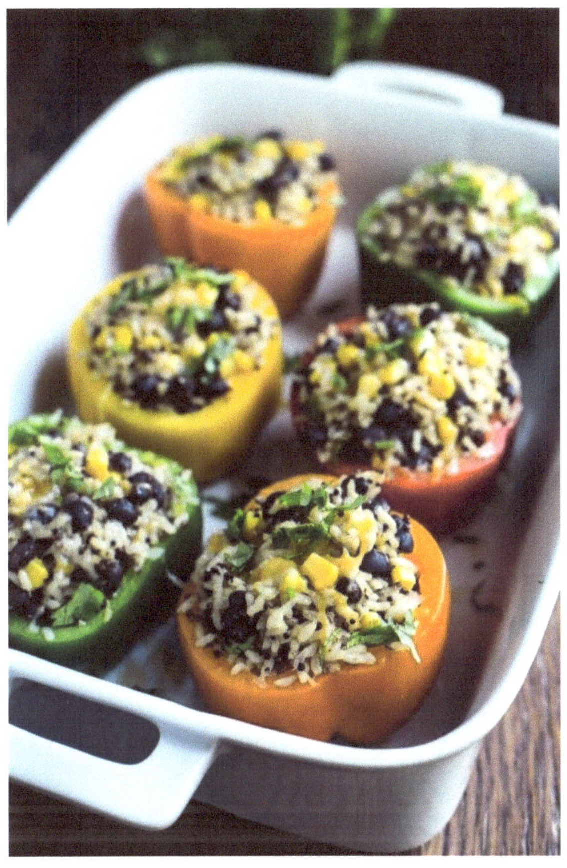

Ingredients

1 ½ Cups Uncooked Brown or White Rice or 2 Packets Brown Rice Quinoa

1 Cup Sweet Corn

1 Can Black Beans

4 Bell Peppers

Vegan Cheese of Choice

Directions

First, lightly grease a baking sheet and pre-heat the oven to 350 degrees.

Cook the rice as directed to do so.

Stir together the black beans and corn. Toss some salt and pepper on and then set it aside.

Cut the tops of the peppers off and tack out the stem and the seeds. Stuff the peppers with the rice and corn mixture.

Place the peppers on the greased sheet and add a little bit of cheese on top of the peppers.

Bake the peppers for about 10 minutes to melt the cheese.

Let it cool and enjoy!

Black Bean Enchiladas

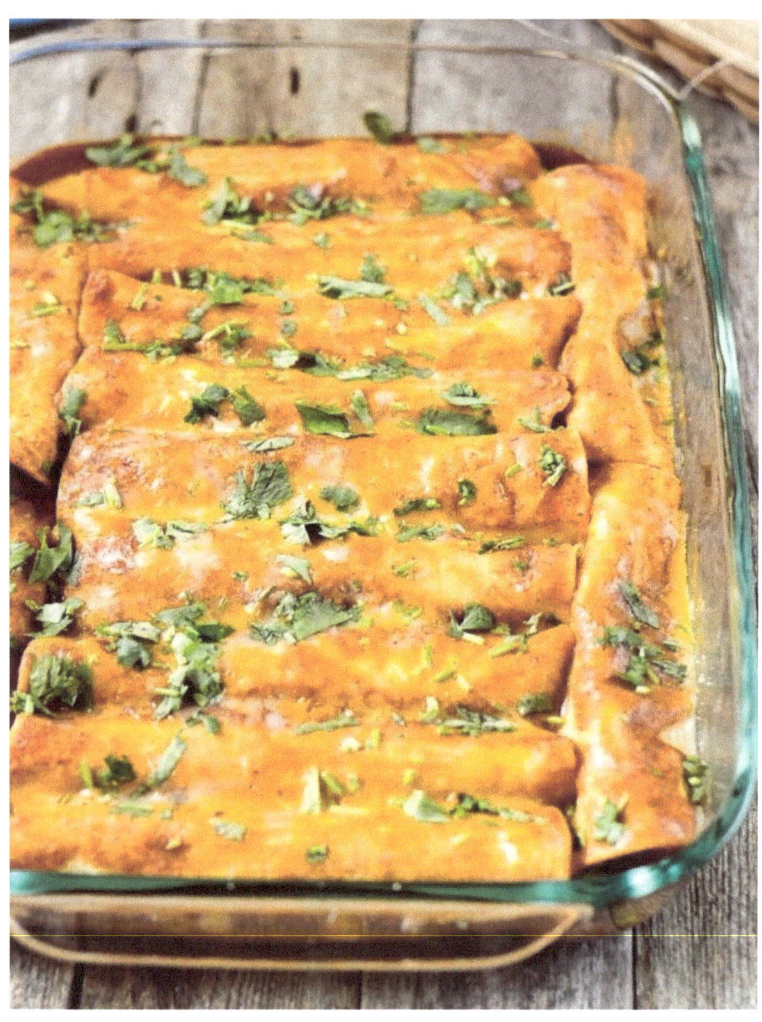

Ingredients

1 Medium Size Yellow Onion

1 Tablespoon Canola Oil

3 Tablespoon Chili Powder

2 Garlic Cloves, Minced

2 Teaspoons Cumin Powder

1 Teaspoons Cooked Black Beans

1 Teaspoon Salt

1 Medium Size Jalapenos

8 Ounces Vegan Cheese

2 Cups Tomato Puree

12-14 (5.5 Inch) Corn Tortillas

Directions

Start out by heating oil in a sauté pan on medium heat. Add onion and garlic and cook for about 3 minutes. Add the cumin powder, chili powder, and salt. Cook for another 2 minutes. Then add the tomato puree and beans. Bring your ingredients to a boil. Turn the heat down to a low temperature. Mash up the beans and let it simmer for 6 minutes.

Afterwards, remove the bean mix from the burner. Strain the ingredients but reserve the sauce. Take the strained bean mixture and place it in a medium bowl. Mix ½ cup cilantro, jalapenos, and 4 ounces of cheese together with the bean mixture.

Preheat the oven to 350 degrees.

Then, spread ½ cup of the sauce in the bottom of a baking dish. Place 5 tortillas in the microwave until softened. Coop ¼ cup of bean mixture into each tortilla. Roll up the tortillas up tightly. Place the filled tortillas in the baking dish with the seam-side facing downward. Pour the remaining sauce over the enchiladas.

Finally, sprinkle the remaining cheese over the enchiladas. Cover the baking dish with aluminum foil and bake for about 20 minutes. Take off the foil and bake for 2-3 minutes until the cheese is slightly brown.

Top the enchiladas with cilantro and serve!

Vegan Pho

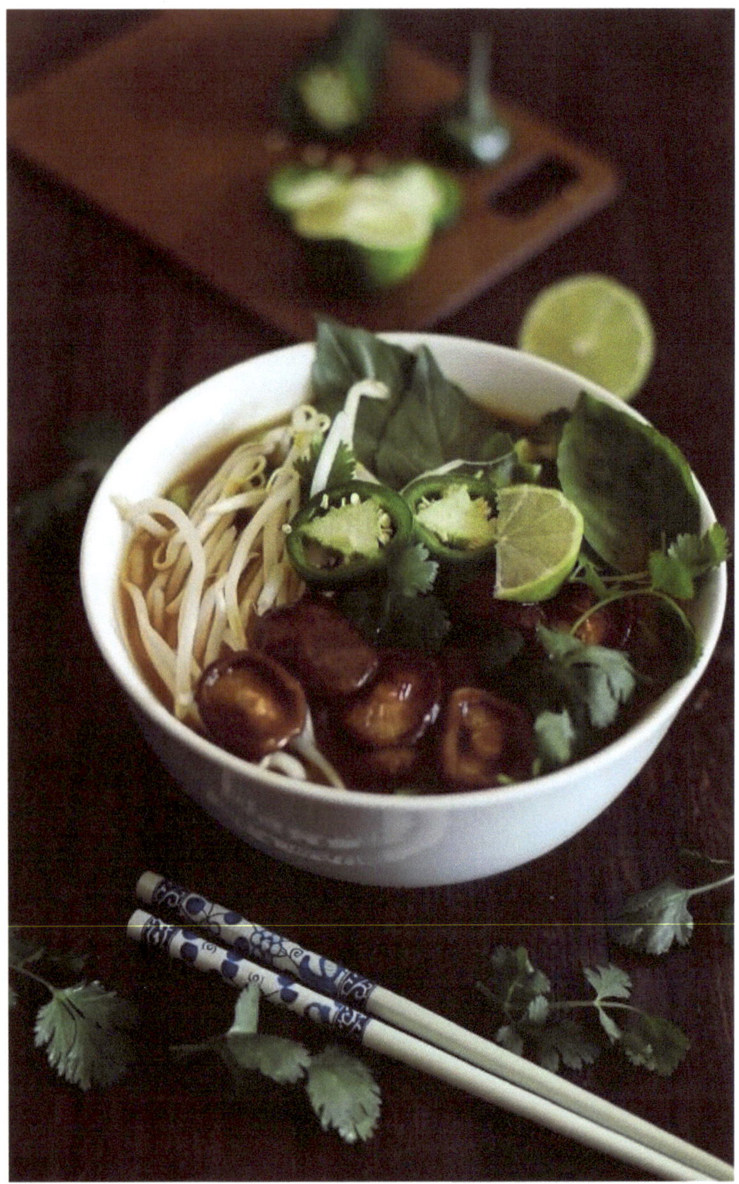

Ingredients

6 Green Onions, Thinly Sliced

1 Tablespoon Fresh Ginger, Peeled and Grated

64 Ounces Homemade Vegetable Broth

1 ½ Tablespoon Butter

6 Ounces Shitake Mushrooms, Remove Stem

2 Teaspoons Sesame Oil

1 ½ Tablespoon Hoisin Sauce

14 Ounces Rice Noodles

2 Jalapeno Peppers, Thinly Sliced

8 Ounces Bean Sprouts

Fresh Basil, Cilantro, Lime wedges, Hoisin Sauce, Sriracha, and chili Garlic Sauce for Serving

Directions

First, combine the vegetable broth, grated ginger, green onion, and salt. Let simmer for 15 minutes.

While the broth cooks, melt the butter in a large skillet over medium heat. Add the mushrooms to the skillet and sauté for about 6 minutes. Stir frequently. Stir in the hoisin and sesame oil. Cook until the sauce thickens. Remove from the heat.

Finally, divide the rice noodles between 4 to 6 bowls. Fill each bowl with the ginger broth. Add sliced jalapenos, shitake mushrooms, bean sprouts, fresh basil, and cilantro. Serve with hoisin, chili garlic sauce, and lime wedges. Enjoy!

Sweet & Spicy Asian Tofu

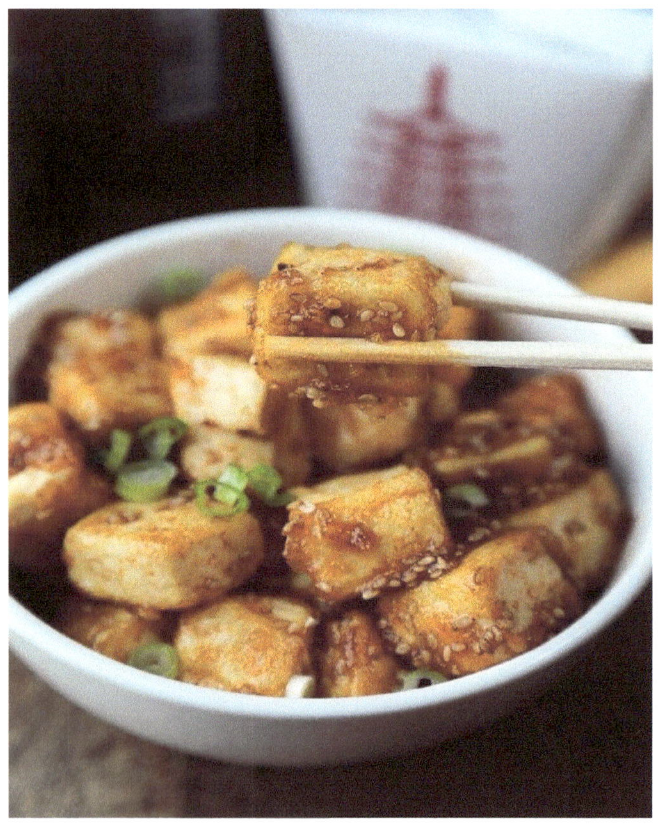

Ingredients

7 Ounces Extra Firm Tofu

1 Garlic Clove, Minced

1 Tablespoon High-Heat Oil

3 Cups Assorted Stir-Fry Vegetables

2 Tablespoons Sriracha Hot Sauce

3 Tablespoons Sweet Chili Sauce

2 Teaspoons Soy Sauce

2/3 Cup Brown Rice

Directions

Before you start cooking, wrap the tofu in paper towels an hour before cooking. Place it between two plates to press out the liquid.

Heat the oil in a pan over medium-high heat. Add the tofu cubes to the hot pan and fry until golden.

Afterwards, set the tofu aside and add some cooking spray to the pan if it's not oily. Sauté the vegetables and garlic over medium-high heat.

As the vegetables and tofu cook, stir together the sauce ingredients. Serve the vegetables and tofu with the brown rice with sauce on top.

Asian Hot Pot

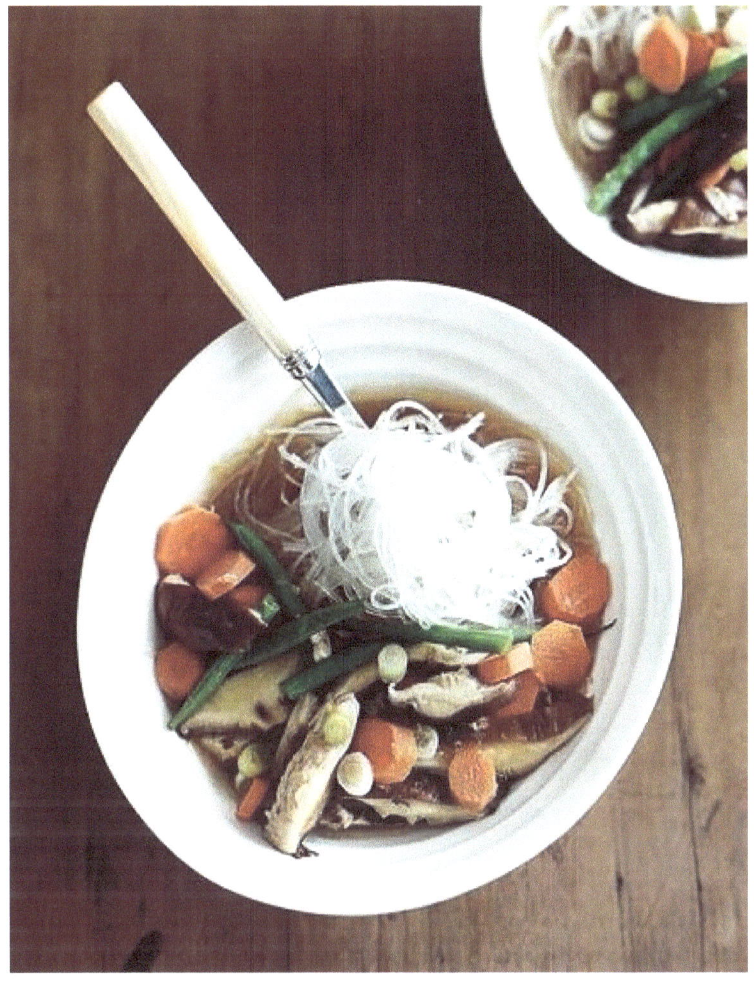

Ingredients

3.75 Ounce Package Cellophane

8 Ounces Shitake Mushrooms

1 Tablespoon Olive Oil

6 Cups Vegetable Broth

2 Tablespoons Grated Fresh Ginger

2/3 Cup Low Sodium Soy Sauce

1 Teaspoon Chili Sauce

4 Carrots, Thinly Sliced

4 Scallions, Thinly Sliced

8 Ounces Green Beans, Trimmed and Cut 2-Inch Pieces

Directions

First, cook the noodles as directed on the package. Drain the noodles and cut into 3 inch lengths.

Afterwards, heat the oil in a large saucepan on medium heat. Add the mushrooms to the pan and cook. Stir the mushrooms for 2 minutes.

Add the soy sauce, broth, and chili sauce and bring to a boil.

Add the carrots, green beans, and scallions. Simmer for about 5 to 6 minutes.

Divide the noodles between a couple bowls and then pour the soup over each one.

Stir Fried Tofu Rice

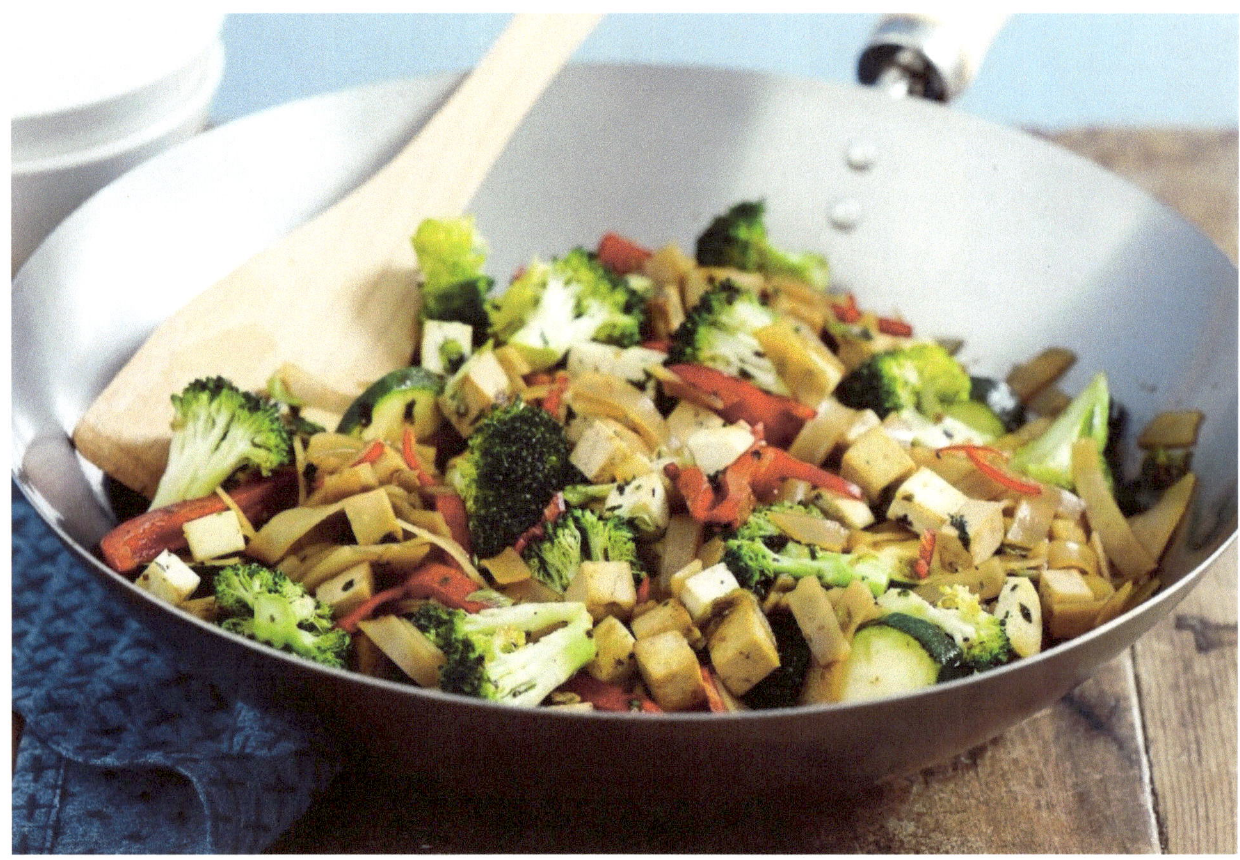

Ingredients

8 Ounce Package Rice Noodles

¼ Cup Low-Sodium Soy Sauce

¼ Cup Brown Sugar

2 Tablespoons Fresh Lime Juice

1 Tablespoon Canola Oil

14 Ounce Package Firm Tofu

2 Carrots, Thinly Cut

Directions

First, boil the noodles as directed on the package and then drain the noodles. Put the noodles back into the pot.

In a small bowl, which together soy sauce, sugar, and lime juice.

Press the tofu slices between paper towels to remove any liquid. Then, cut the tofu into ½ inch pieces.

Pour the oil in a large skillet and place it on medium-high heat. Add the bell pepper, carrots, and ginger. Stir the ingredients for 2 minutes. Add the bean sprouts and tofu. Cook and stir until the vegetables

1 Red Bell Pepper, Thinly Sliced

2 Cups Bean Sprouts

1 Tablespoon Grated Fresh Ginger

4 Scallion, Thinly Sliced

¼ Cup Roasted Peanuts, Roughly Chopped

are slightly tender, which would be about 3 to 4 minutes.

Then, toss the noodles in half the soy sauce mixture and cook over medium heat for 1 to 2 minutes. Pour the vegetable mixture and the soy sauce mixture on the noodles.

Finally, sprinkle with peanuts, scallions, and cilantro. Enjoy!

Vegan Pizza

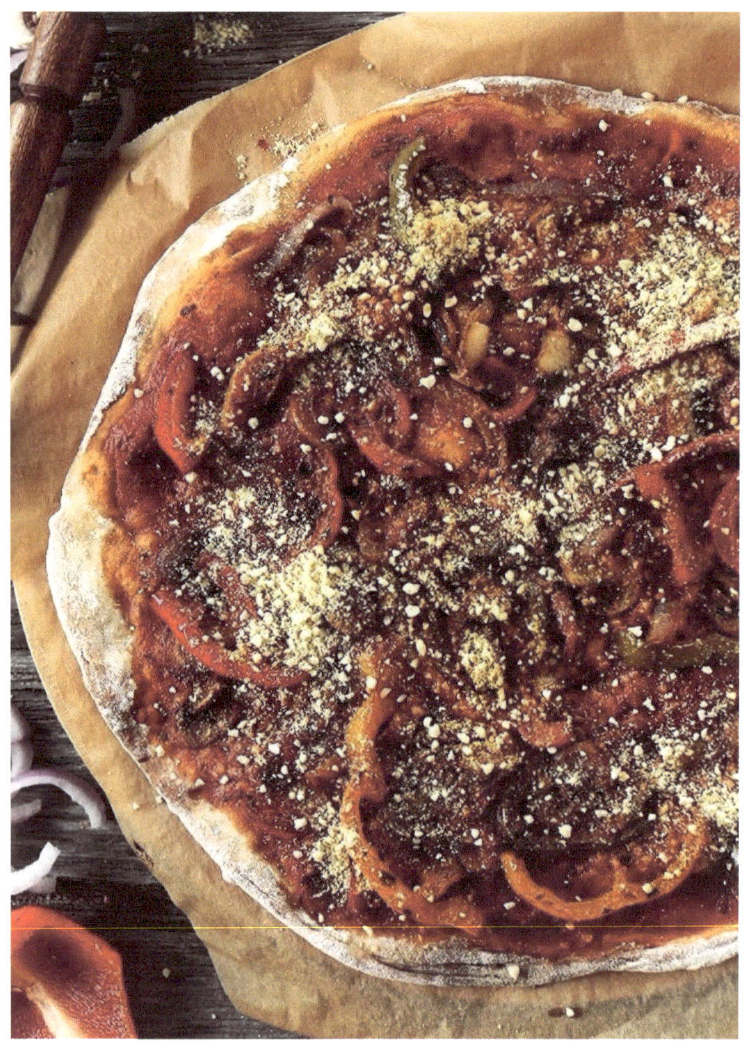

Ingredients

½ Trader Joe's Garlic-Herb Pizza Crust

1/3 Cup Red Onion, Chopped

½ Cup Each Red, Green, and Orange Bell Pepper, Loosely Chopped

1 Cup Button Mushrooms, Chopped

¼ Teaspoon Sea alt

½ Teaspoons Each Dried Fresh Basil, Oregano, and Garlic Powder

15 Ounce Can Tomato Sauce

¼ Teaspoon Sea Salt

1/2 Cup Vegan Parmesan Cheese

Red Pepper Flake and Dried Oregano

Directions

Preheat the oven to 425 degrees F.

Place a large skillet over medium heat. Add 1 Tablespoon of olive oil, onion, and peppers to the hot skillet. Season with salt and herbs, and then stir. Cook for about 10 to 15 minutes and then add the mushrooms during the last few minutes.

You can prepare the sauce by adding tomato sauce to a mixing bowl. Add seasonings and salt to the bowl.

Prepare the vegan parmesan by blitzing raw cashes, nutritional yeast, sea salt, and garlic powder in a blender. Take this mixture and pour it into a jar, and set it in the refrigerator.

Roll out the dough onto a floured surface. Then, take the dough and place it on a a round baking sheet with parchment paper.

Top the dough with as much sauce as you'd prefer. Then sprinkle the parmesan cheese and the sautéed veggies.

Gently slid the pizza with the parchment sheet only (Not the pan) on the oven rack.

Bake the pizza for 17 to 20 minutes or until golden brown.

Serve with the remaining dried oregano, red pepper flake, and parmesan cheese. Enjoy!

Cauliflower Pizza

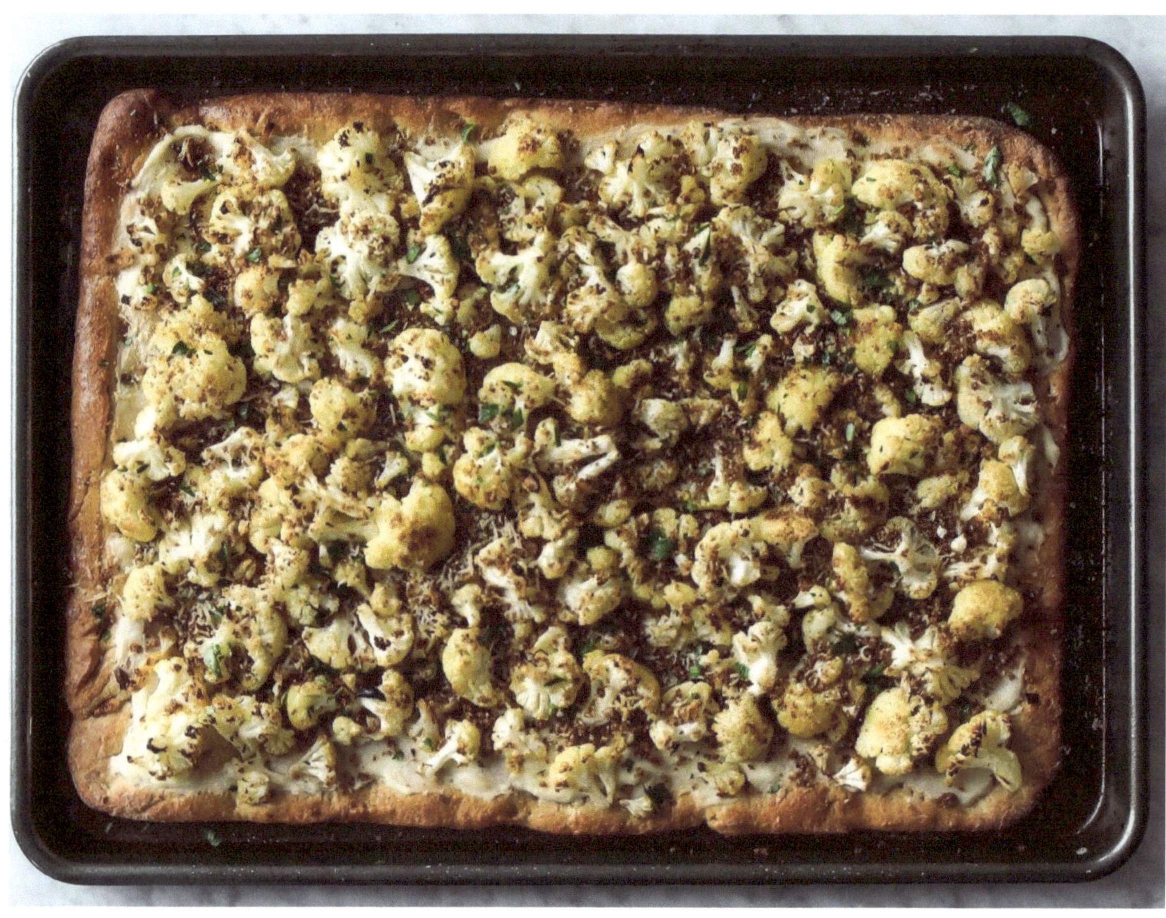

Ingredients

4 Cups Cauliflower Florets

1 ½ Teaspoon Salt

¼ Cup Extra Virgin Olive Oil

½ Teaspoon Ground Black Pepper

1 Recipe Thin Crust Pizza Dough

Cornmeal

Flour

Directions

First, Mix the cauliflower florets, salt, ground pepper, and extra virgin olive oil together in a bowl.

Roast the cauliflower on a baking pan at 400 degrees for about 20 minutes.

Roll out your pizza dough on a floured 12 by 16-inch rectangle. Then, place the dough on a cornmeal-dusted baking pan.

Top the dough with the cauliflower and breadcrumbs.

Bake the pizza at 500 degrees until golden. This

3 Tablespoon Breadcrumbs

should take about 15 minutes.

Place on a cutting board and serve!

Italian Orzo Spinach Soup

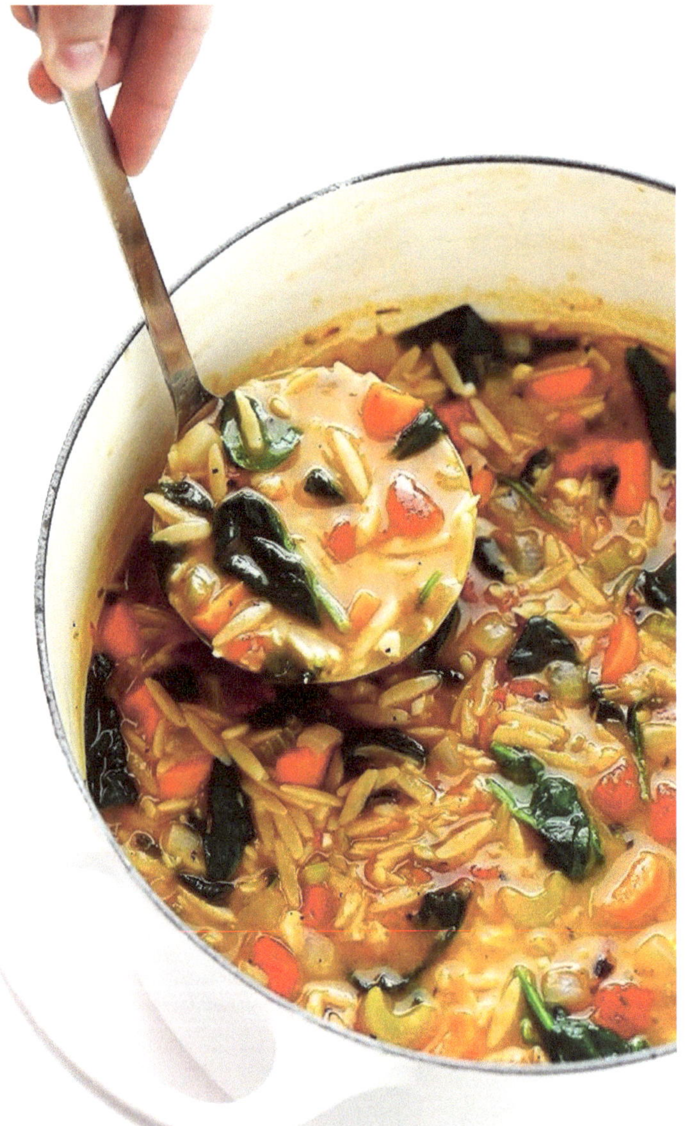

Ingredients

1 Small White Onion, Peeled and Diced

1 Tablespoons Olive Oil

1 Cup Diced Carrots

3 Garlic Cloves, Peeled and Minced

1 Cup Diced Celery

6 Cups Chicken Stock

14 Ounce Can Dire-Roasted Diced Tomatoes

1 ½ Cups DeLallo Whole Wheat Orzo Pasta

¼ Teaspoon Dried Oregano

½ Teaspoon Dried Thyme

¼ Teaspoon Dried Rosemary

4 Cups Loosely-Packed Spinach

Salt and Black Pepper

Directions

Start out by heating oil in a large stock pot over medium-high temperature. Add onion and sauté for 4 minutes. Add carrots, garlic, and celery; sauté for another 3 minutes.

Then, add chicken stock, orzo, tomatoes, thyme, rosemary, oregano, and stir. Bring the soup to a simmer for 10 minutes. Stir the soup occasionally.

Stir in the spinach and cook for about 1-2 minutes. Season your soup with salt and black pepper.

Serve and enjoy!

Winter Lentil Soup

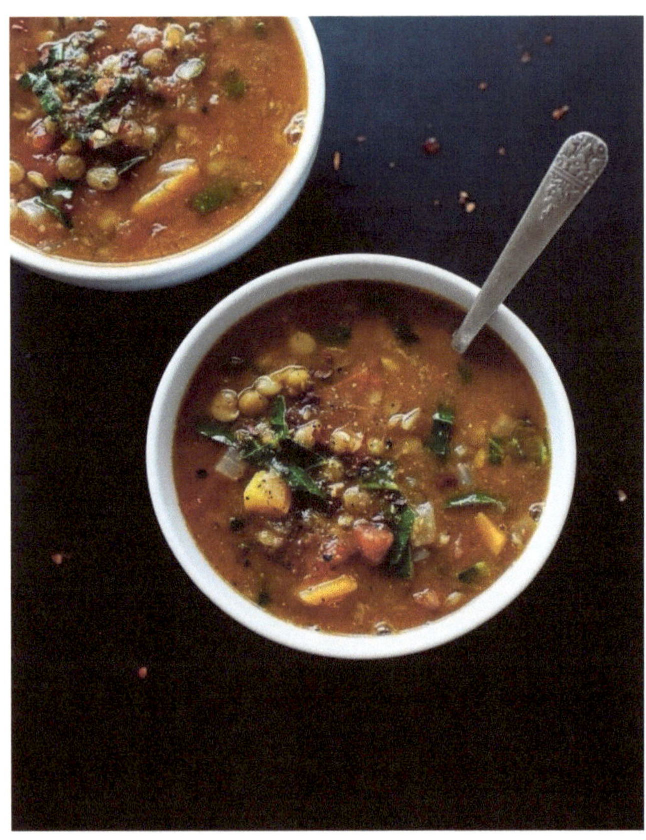

Ingredients

4 Leeks, Cut ¼ Inch Thick Half Moons

1 Tablespoon Olive Oil

28 Ounce Can Whole Tomatoes, drained

2 Sweet Potatoes, Peeled and Cut ½ Inch Pieces

½ Cup Brown Lentils

1 Tablespoon Fresh Thyme

1 Bunch Kale, Stems Removed and Leaves Cut ½ Inch Wide Strips

Kosher Salt and Black Pepper

Directions

First, heat the oil in a large heavy bottom pot over medium heat. Add the leeks and stir occasionally for about 3 to 4 minutes. Add the tomatoes and cook. Stir every 5 minutes.

Add 6 cups of water and bring the pot to a boil. Pour in the sweet potatoes, lentils, kale, thyme, ¼ teaspoon pepper, and 1 ½ teaspoon salt. Simmer until the lentils are tender. This should take about 25 to 30 minutes.

Pour into bowls and enjoy!

Chickpea Red Pepper Soup

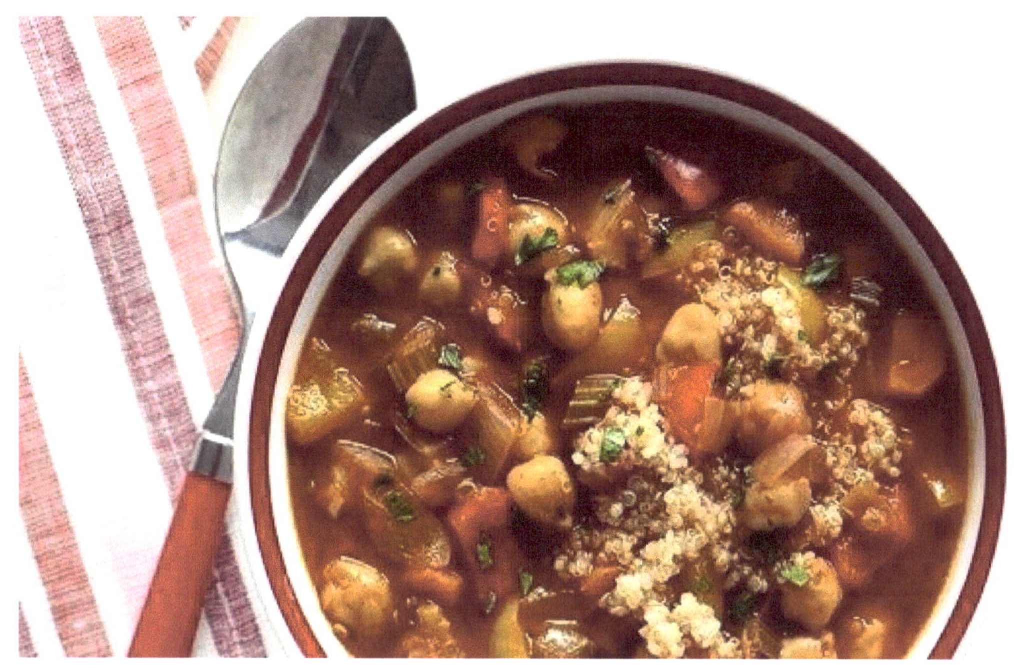

Ingredients

2 Tablespoon Olive Oil

½ Quinoa

1 Carrot

3 Garlic Cloves

2 Celery Stalks

1 Tablespoon Smoked Paprika

Kosher Salt

Pepper

1 Red Pepper

Directions

First, cook the quinoa according to package.

Heat the oil in a large heavy-bottomed pot. Add the onion, celery, and carrot. Cook the ingredients, cover the pot, and stir every 6 minutes.

Add paprika, garlic, and ¼ teaspoon of salt and pepper. Stir for 1 minute. Add the peppers and continue to cook. Stir every 5 minutes.

Add the chickpeas, 1 cup of water, and broth. Bring the pot to a boil. Reduce the heat to a simmer. Cook for about 5 to 8 minutes. Stir in the vinegar and cooked quinoa.

Serve with parsley on top.

1 Yellow

2 Can Low Sodium Chickpeas

1 Tablespoon Red wine Vinegar

2 Cups Low Sodium Vegetable Broth

Chopped Fresh Parsley

Conclusion

Thank you for reading our vegan cook book. Hopefully it was interesting and it served you well. If you're a beginner and are considering picking up the vegan diet, then I wish you the best. Enjoy these delicious recipes. Please leave a review on Amazon. We'd really appreciate hearing your feedback.

Work Cited

"30-Minute Vegetarian Pho Recipe." *Oh My Veggies*, 15 May 2014, https://ohmyveggies.com/30-minute-vegetarian-pho/.

"Avocado Pasta." *Damn Delicious*, 4 Nov. 2016, http://damndelicious.net/2014/06/20/avocado-pasta/.

"Black Bean Vegan Enchiladas." *Light Orange Bean*, 7 Jan. 2017, https://lightorangebean.com/black-bean-vegan-enchiladas/.

"List of Foods That Vegans Eat." *Healthy Eating | SF Gate*, www.healthyeating.sfgate.com/list-foods-vegans-eat-3763.html.

"Recipe: Vegetarian Paella with Red Peppers & Chickpeas." *Kitchn*, www.thekitchn.com/recipe-vegetable-paella-recipes-from-the-kitchn-216585.

86lemons.Com, https://86lemons.com/amazing-veggie-quesadillas/.

Alina, et al. "Vegan Zucchini 'Meatballs'." *Making Thyme for Health*, 28 Feb. 2017, http://makingthymeforhealth.com/vegan-zucchini-meatballs/#comments.

Baker, Minimalist, et al. "Simple Vegan Pizza | Minimalist Baker Recipes." *Minimalist Baker*, 27 June 2017, https://minimalistbaker.com/my-favorite-vegan-pizza/.

Baker, Minimalist, et al. "Vegan Fajitas | Minimalist Baker Recipes." *Minimalist Baker*, 29 June 2017, https://minimalistbaker.com/poblano-and-portobello-fajitas/.

Baker, Minimalist, et al. "Vegan Green Chili Mac n Cheese | Minimalist Baker Recipes." *Minimalist Baker*, 28 June 2017, www.minimalistbaker.com/vegan-green-chili-mac-n-cheese/.

Britnell, B. "Burrito Bowl Stuffed Peppers." *B. Britnell*, 10 Aug. 2016, http://bbritnell.com/burrito-bowl-stuffed-peppers/.

Chun, Kay. "Pasta With Green Olive Pesto." *Real Simple*, 1 Aug. 2003, www.realsimple.com/food-recipes/browse-all-recipes/pasta-green-olive-pesto-10000000524318/index.html.

Farley, Jennifer. "Sweet and Spicy Asian Tofu." *Savory Simple*, 19 Mar. 2016, www.savorysimple.net/spicy-asian-tofu-weight-watchers/.

Kitchen, Food Network. "Vegan Lemon Fettuccine Alfredo." *Food Network*, Food Network, 4 Mar. 2014, www.foodnetwork.com/recipes/food-network-kitchen/vegan-lemon-fettuccine-alfredo-3362345.

Merker, Kate. "Stir-Fried Rice Noodles With Tofu and Vegetables." *Real Simple*, 1 Sept. 2009,
    www.realsimple.com/food-recipes/browse-all-recipes/stir-fried-rice-noodles-tofu-vegetables-
    00000000019604/index.html.

Nicholson, Cynthia. "Black Beans and Rice." *Real Simple*, 1 Feb. 2005, www.realsimple.com/food-
    recipes/browse-all-recipes/black-beans-rice-10000001031604/index.html.

Oven, Gimme Some. "Italian Orzo Spinach Soup." *Gimme Some Oven*, 24 Apr. 2017,
    www.gimmesomeoven.com/italian-orzo-spinach-soup-recipe/.

Quessenberry, Sara. "Asian Hot Pot." *Real Simple*, 1 Feb. 2007, www.realsimple.com/food-recipes/browse-
    all-recipes/asian-hot-pot.

Quessenberry, Sara. "Winter Lentil Soup." *Real Simple*, 1 Mar. 2006, www.realsimple.com/food-
    recipes/browse-all-recipes/winter-lentil-soup-10000001151425/index.html.

Smith, Art. "Chickpea and Red Pepper Soup with Quinoa." *Country Living*, 11 Aug. 2016,
    www.countryliving.com/food-drinks/recipes/a34596/chickpea-red-pepper-soup-quinoa-recipe-
    wdy0214/.

Unknown. "Roasted Cauliflower Pizza." *Country Living*, 14 Sept. 2015, www.countryliving.com/food-
drinks/recipes/a4273/roasted-cauliflower-pizza-recipe-clv0108/